For Sarah and Benjamin
J.W.

For George
T.W.

LITTLE TIGER PRESS
An imprint of Magi Publications
1 The Coda Centre, 189 Munster Road, London SW6 6AW
www.littletigerpress.com

First published in Great Britain 1999
This edition published 2005

Have you got my Purr?

by
Judy West and Tim Warnes

LITTLE TIGER PRESS
London

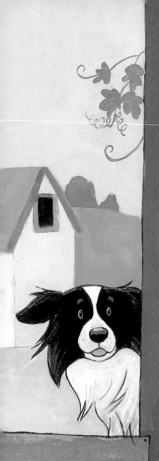

"Oh Mummy, Mummy!"

"What's the matter, little Kitten?
Why are you crying?"

"Oh Mummy, Mummy, I've lost my purr.

"You'll find your purr, little Kitten.
Just wait and see."

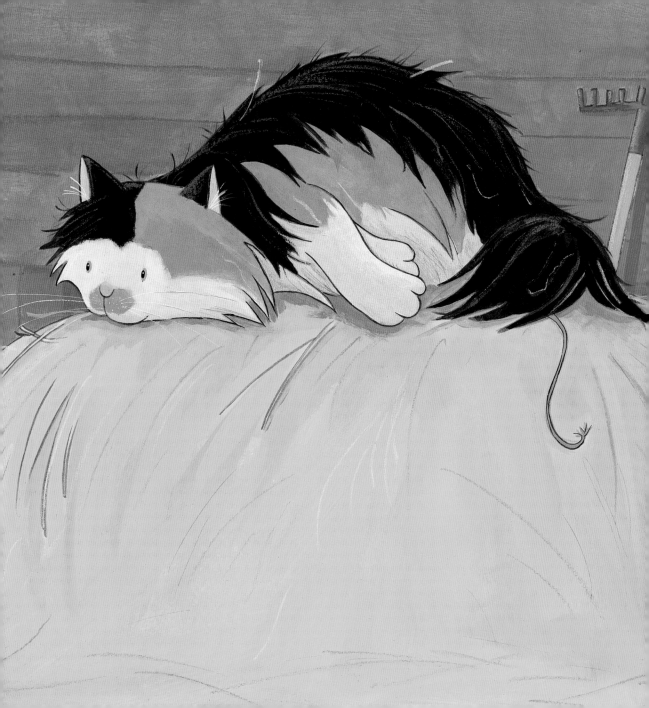

"Oh Dog, Dog, have you got my purr?"
"Woof, woof," said Dog, licking his bone.
"I haven't got your purr, little Kitten.
This is my *woof*. Why don't you ask Cow?"

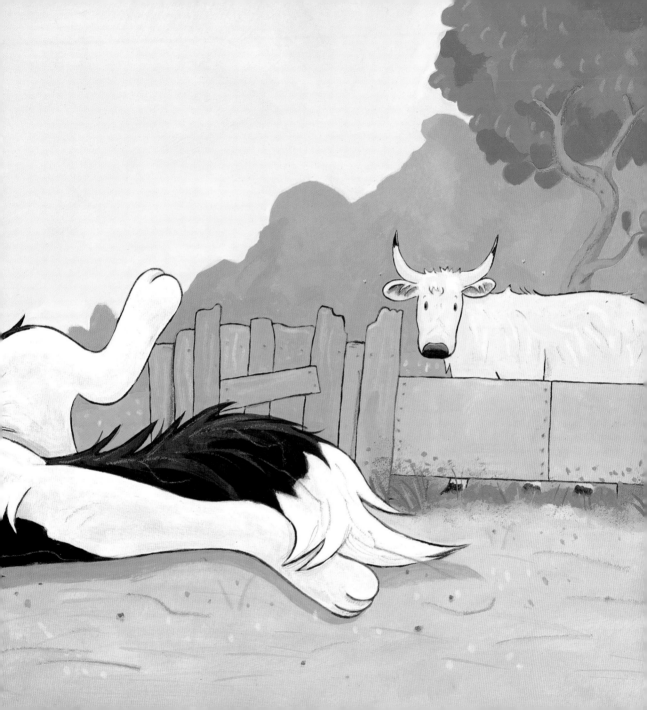

"Oh Cow, Cow, have
you got my purr?"
"Moo, moo," said Cow,
flicking flies with
her ears.

MOO

MOO

"I haven't got your purr,
little Kitten. This is my *moo*.
Why don't you ask Pig?"

"Oh Pig, Pig, have you got my purr?"
"Oink, oink," said Pig, snuffling
in the straw.

OINK
OINK

"I haven't got your purr, little Kitten. This is my *oink*. Why don't you ask Duck?"

"Oh Duck, Duck, have you
got my purr?"
"Quack, quack," said Duck,
splashing in the water.

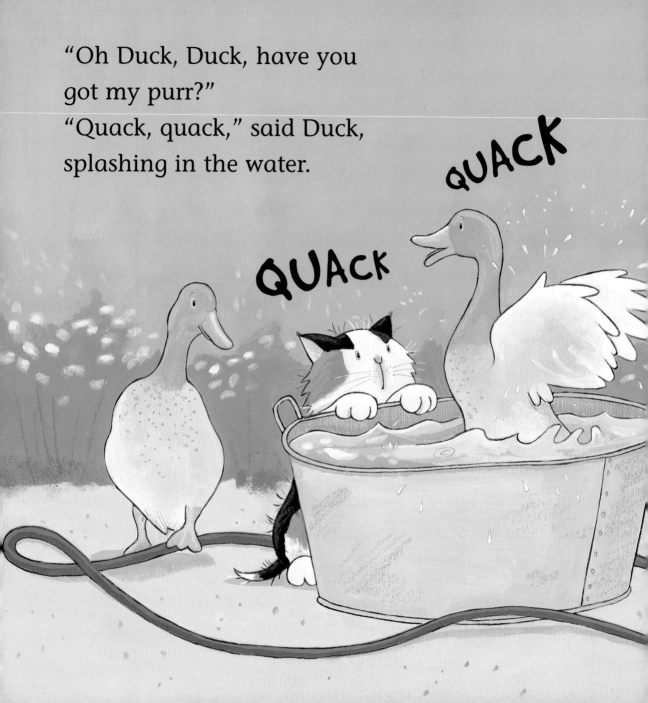

"I haven't got your purr, little Kitten. This is my *quack*. Why don't you ask Mouse?"

"Oh Mouse, Mouse, have you got my purr?"
"Squeak, squeak," said Mouse, nibbling cheese
in the barn. "I haven't got your purr, little Kitten.
This is my *squeak*. Why don't you ask Sheep?"

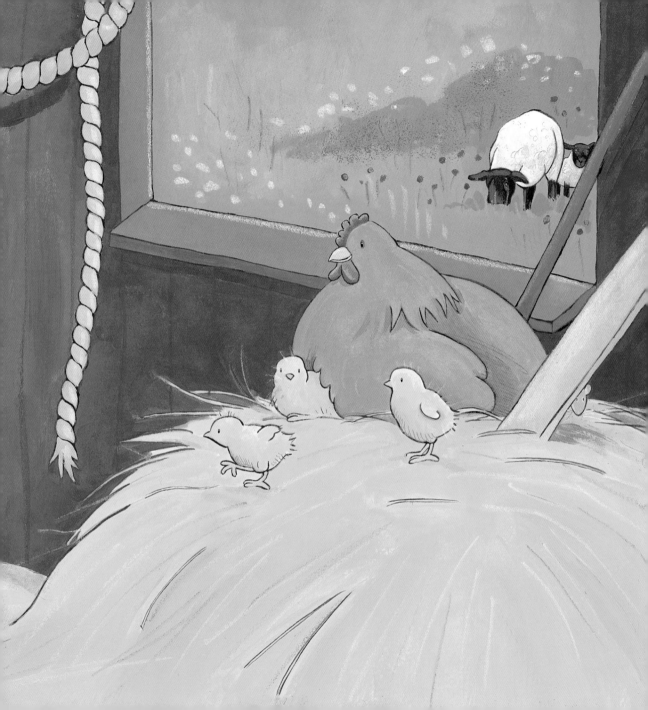

"Oh Sheep, Sheep, have you got my purr?"
"Baa, baa," said Sheep, munching grass in
the field. "I haven't got your purr, little Kitten.
This is my *baa*. Why don't you ask wise old Owl?"

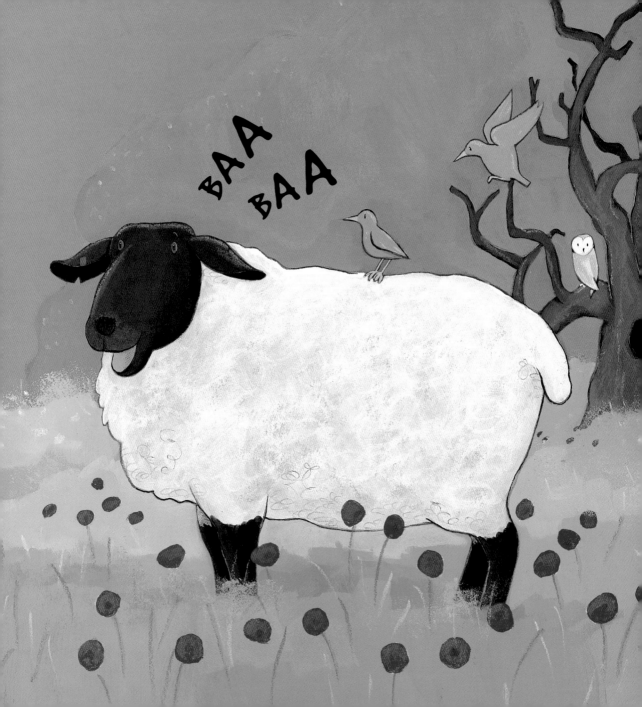

"Wise old Owl, have you got my purr?"
"Hoot, hoot," said the wise old Owl, blinking his big round eyes.

HOOT
HOOT

"I haven't got your purr, little Kitten.
This is my *hoot*. Why don't you go
back and ask your mother?"

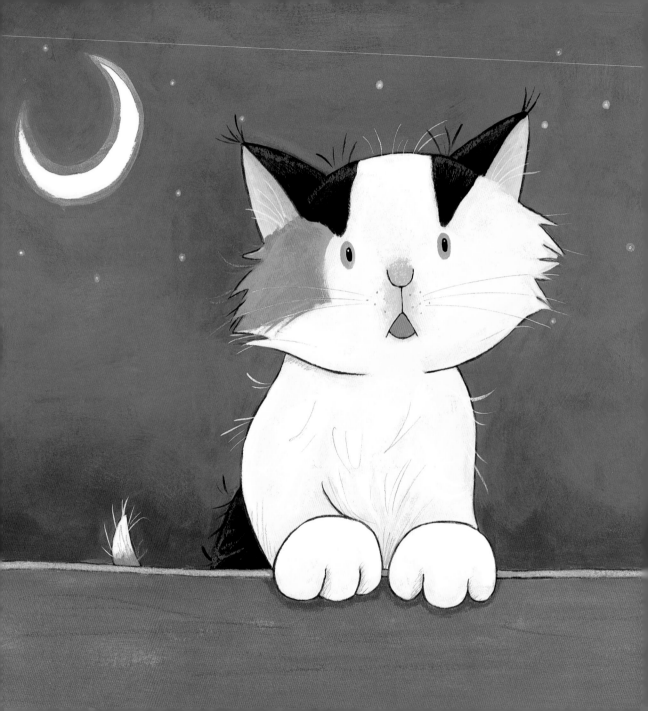

"Oh Mummy, Mummy," wailed little Kitten. "*Nobody's* got my purr. Dog hasn't got it. He's got a woof. Cow hasn't got it. She's got a moo. Pig hasn't got it. She's got an oink. Duck hasn't got it. She's got a quack. Mouse hasn't got it. He's got a squeak. Sheep hasn't got it. She's got a baa. Wise old Owl hasn't got it. He's got a hoot. Oh Mummy, Mummy, I've lost my purr!"

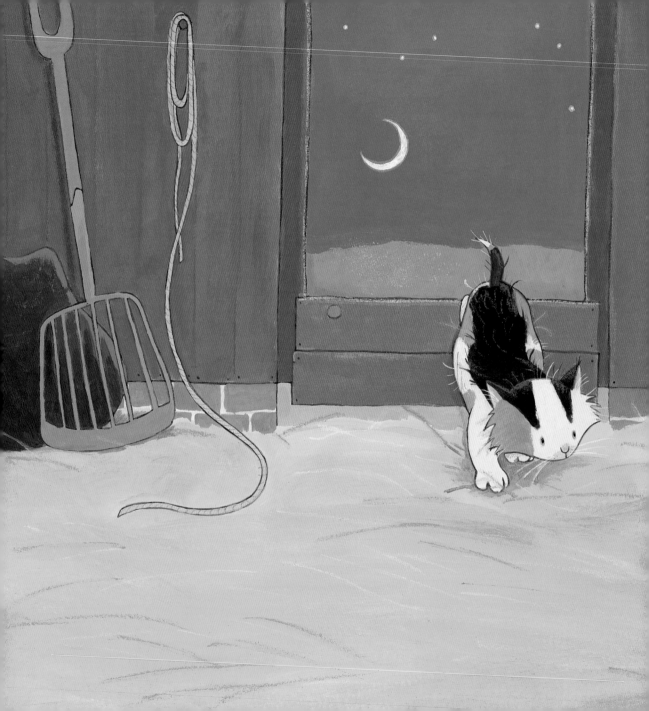

"You haven't lost your purr,
little Kitten. Come here
and I'll explain.

"Nobody's got your purr.
Your purr is inside you
when you're happy!
Listen, little Kitten,
listen . . ."

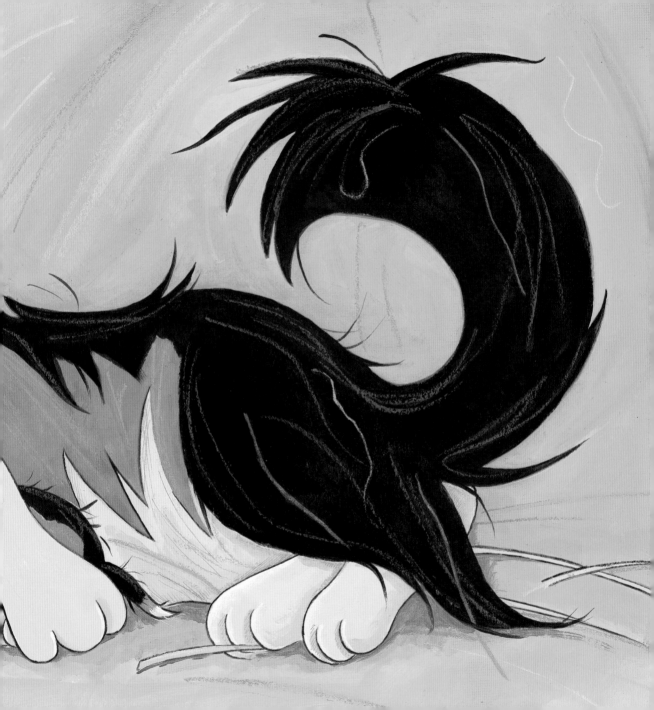

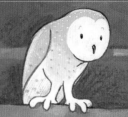

"My *purr!*
Oh, Mummy.
I've found my purr!
It was here
all the time."
So little Kitten
curled up . . .

and purred and purred
and purred.

PURR PURR

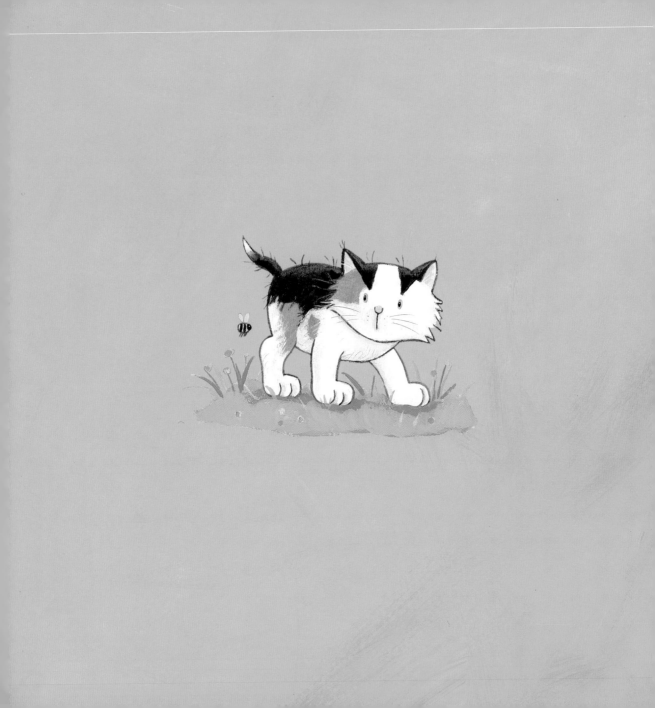